TAKE CHARGE OF YOUR HEALTH

Live to be 100 by Healing Yourself Naturally

By Tammy Moore

Legal & Disclaimer

The information contained in this book is not designed to replace or take the place of any form of medicine or professional medical advice. The information in this book has been provided for educational and entertainment purposes only.

The information contained in this book has been compiled from sources deemed reliable, and it is accurate to the best of the Author's knowledge; however, the Author cannot guarantee its accuracy and validity and cannot be held liable for any errors or omissions. Changes are periodically made to this book. You must consult your doctor or get professional medical advice before using any of the suggested remedies, techniques, or information in this book.

Upon using the information contained in this book, you agree to hold harmless the Author from and against any damages, costs, and expenses, including any legal fees potentially resulting from the application of any of the information provided by this guide. This disclaimer applies to any damages or injury caused by the use and application, whether directly or indirectly, of any advice or information presented, whether for breach of contract, tort, negligence, personal injury, criminal intent, or under any other cause of action.

You agree to accept all risks of using the information presented inside this book. You need to consult a professional medical practitioner in order to ensure you are both able and healthy enough to participate in this program.

Table of Contents

Introduction

The term "personalized medicine" has created quite a buzz recently. It refers to the concept of people taking charge of their own health, managing it with the use of technologies like iPhone ECGs, personal genomes, and the diverse array of information that can be obtained from the internet.

Instead of consulting a doctor for that chronic headache or constant pain in the back, people can search the web to look for symptoms similar to their own, do a self-diagnosis, and then make use of home remedies that pertain to their condition.

There's no scientific proof that this method of healthcare works. Some argue that it's unsafe, putting a person's health and wellbeing at risk. However, many who have tried home remedies feel assured that they are effective, and that they have saved them hundreds or even thousands of dollars from hospital or doctor's fees.

This is just one of the many aspects to consider when managing your own health. It's imperative to weigh the pros and cons in order to make an informed decision.

I was motivated to write this book due to my own personal experience. I had an extended fever (for more than a week) and I went to see the doctor and I was hospitalized. I stayed in the hospital for 5-days, the doctors ran many expensive tests, and the bill was quite expensive. They told me I had cancer, and send me to a cancer center as part of the nearby university. They wanted to run more invasive tests and start treatment right away. At this point I started to feel a bit better, and I just could not believe I had cancer (I know no one believes they have cancer), and I refuse to run the additional tests, at least not that day. So I went home, much to the fear and disappointment of my spouse. He felt that I was in denial and wanted me to run those tests and start treatment. That evening a friend came to visit me, and she sided with my husband. To keep the peace, she suggested we get a second opinion. It was the best advice of our lives. We went to a private cancer center who spoke with an infectious disease doctor. A few less invasive tests were suggested to better diagnose my ailment. At the same time we read books and searched the internet in case it was cancer. We started to eat super healthy, juiced 3-4 times a day, and waited to get an updated from the new tests. Well, I was right I had mononucleosis (mono for short),

2

something we asked the Doctor about in the Hospital. The mono-spot test used for mono is considered to be only ~55% accurate and depends on the stage the virus is at when they run the test. The new healthy eating and juicing made me get stronger week by week, and as is the case with most viruses your body has to fight it on its own. Thanks to the new healthy lifestyle I was back on my feet in a few more weeks.

What I learned from that experience is what my Aunt had been showing me and telling me for years. She always ate healthy, stayed active, minimized how much red meat she ate, never smoked, and rarely drank alcohol. I should have listened all of those years!!

I hope you enjoy the book and the tips I have learned from my personal experiences.

Pros and Cons of Self-Healthcare

On the side of the advantages, you'll find the following items are good reasons to manage your own health:

- Personalized – No one knows you better than yourself. A doctor whom you've just met will probe your background down to your childhood but even so, it won't be enough for him to know your body the same way that you do. It's you who have spent years getting to know the ins and outs of your health. Often, you will feel when you go to visit a doctor that he wants to get you out as quickly as possible and collect some money. He may not take the time to hear all the symptoms of your issue, and ready to write you a prescription and get you out the door.

- Less expensive – Doctor's fees, hospital bills, and medications can all add up. If your budget doesn't allow it, you're not going to get the treatment that you need. Your health insurance may help a little but it still can get expensive. With all your regular monthly expenses, you just can't afford any additional bills.

- More natural and less invasive – When you decide to care for your own health, you'll be using natural remedies that are not only safe but also less invasive. Many feel that using natural remedies can also build a better immune system and make your body more prepared for those unexpected illnesses when you do have them. You may not even know when you have some minor illnesses as your body's immune system is so well protected.

- Availability of information – Today, there is plenty of credible information that can be found online. If you need medical information, reputable medical websites are easily found. You just have to be vigilant in your research. Don't believe everything that you see on the internet. See to it that either medical experts have written the information or that you verify it with a few different independent websites.

There are some disadvantages that you need to consider when deciding to become your own doctor

- Unsafe – Yes, it's true that becoming your own doctor can take on some risk. It's possible to put your health at risk taking remedies and medications that your doctor did not prescribe. This is why, it's important to rely on home remedies initially, only for minor ailments. You should read up carefully especially information regarding "when to see your doctor". On the other hand, one can also read about doctors who have incorrectly prescribed medication or where people spend all they have to care for a loved one only to lose them. In emergency situations like broken bones or serious cuts one should rely on Emergency room doctor care, and not try to do it yourself if you are not trained.

- Complicated – Diagnosis is one of the most complicated aspects of medical care. It's because of the spectrum of diseases that are so diverse and most are overlapping in signs and symptoms that you might never really figure out what's wrong with you unless you go see your doctor. Although, I have experienced the case where I did see a doctor and he diagnosed me wrong and I was able to do research get a second opinion and correctly diagnose myself. So do your homework when it comes to complicated diseases.

So what do you think? Are you ready to become the boss of your own health? Let this book be your guide to self-healthcare. It won't tell you to completely shun medical advice as you're going to need it at some point in your life. Instead, it will advise you how to minimize visits to the doctor by leading a healthy and active lifestyle, making use of tried-and-tested remedies for simple and minor ailments, and doing your own research while getting second or third opinions from doctors for serious unknown ailments.

Chapter 1 – Consulting Your Doctor

Asking Your Doctor the Right Questions

Doctors see dozens of people every day. It's no wonder you might feel that your checkup is rushed. It's as if you're not getting the care and attention you need from your doctor. To help avoid such scenarios, prepare for your doctor's appointment so that you'll be able to ask the right questions to help yourself with your diagnosis.

General Questions about Overall Health

What do I need to do to improve my general health & strengthen my immune system?

Your checkup is the perfect time to discuss with your doctor your basic vital statistics. It's also a great idea to talk to him/her about your personal health goals. Do you want to reduce stress levels? Do you plan to become more physically active? Do you want to lose weight? Discuss any of these matters so that your doctor can advise the right kind of diet, exercise and lifestyle changes that you need.

What is this medical test for? What are the risks and benefits?

If your doctor suggests performing any medical examination, you need to know first what why it is needed and what risks and benefits come with it. A survey conducted by the American Board of Internal Medicine Foundation states that almost 75 percent of doctors in the United States perform unnecessary medical examinations. Discussing medical tests with your doctor instead of just passively accepting everything that is suggested for you is the first step in taking an active role in your personal health.

Is this medication necessary for my condition? What are its side effects?

Don't hesitate to ask your doctor about the medications prescribed to you. Feel free to inquire about its side effects. It would also be a good idea to show your doctor the current medications that you're taking so he/she will know if there are any possible interactions between the drugs. If you have any allergies, be sure to inform your physician.

Other Questions to Ask Your Doctor

About your current ailment or diagnosis

- Why do you think I have this condition?

- What tests helped you isolate the disease?

- How might this condition affect my work and family life?

- What is the disease's short-term and long-term prognosis?

- Will I be needing follow up tests or checkups?

- How will this disease be controlled or treated?

About your treatment method

- What are my options in terms of treatment?

- What are the pros and cons of each treatment?

- How much is the suggested treatment?

- How long will each treatment option take?

- Which treatment is most effective for my condition?

- What are the side effects of the treatment?

- What will happen if I don't get treatment or if I delay treatment?

- Will my job or life be affected by the treatment?

Getting a Second or Third Opinion

Even if you have done everything you can to make sure you've chosen a reputable and qualified doctor, there might still come a time that you'll have some doubts about his/her diagnosis, or even his/her expertise on your health matters. If this is the case, you might feel comfortable getting a second or third opinion, especially when it comes to sensitive or serious medical issues.

It's normal to be a little hesitant at first, as you might think that questioning your doctor's credibility or authority is a form of "betrayal" on your part. Especially if you've already gotten close to your doctor, it is normal for us to believe that doctors are experts or should be smarter than you are. It is important to remember that it is your health and life at stake. If your doctor is a true professional she will welcome a patient's request for second or third opinion, and should not feel threaten by such an inquiry.

When to Consult another Doctor

Feel free to get second or third opinion in the following situations:

- You have a serious or potentially fatal disease

- The treatment advised by the doctor sounds risky

- The assessed diagnosis is not clear to you

- The treatment being proposed to you sounds expensive or has had limited success in the past

Tips for Getting Second or Third Opinion

- Talk to your doctor about it. Here's one way to inform your doctor: "I respect your credibility and expertise but my family feels more comfortable if I can seek a second opinion just to be sure about this matter."

- Do your research. Don't just ask the next doctor that you encounter. The amount of time and effort you spent looking for your first doctor should be the same for the doctor you're going to ask a second opinion from.

- Bring all your medical history. Be sure to show the new doctor copies of all medical exams, blood tests, scans and other treatment methods that you've had. He/she will need all the information he/she can get in coming up with an accurate diagnosis of the condition that you have. Most doctors will not challenge a previous diagnosis initially, so be prepared to ask all the same questions to the second doctor as well.

- Plan for the next steps. After you get a second opinion, it will take some time to consider all your options. Do you feel more comfortable going through with the treatment proposed by your new doctor, or the one suggested by the first doctor? If you still do not feel satisfied you can & should consider a third opinion. Initial consultations are less expensive than many medical diagnosis or treatments, so ask as many doctors as you feel you need to.

Western Medical Practices Linked to Pharmaceutical Businesses

How Western Medical Practices that appear tied to Pharmaceutical Businesses

When your doctor prescribes you medication, do you ever wonder or ask if there's a natural treatment option that you could try instead?

A lot of people would probably say "no"—which isn't surprising because a lot of people have come to trust their doctors implicitly and do as they are told. After all, Western medicine is big on effectiveness and safety protocols. Every new drug or treatment is tested rigorously and studied extensively before being granted a stamp of approval. So why worry?

As it turns out, however, this process does not guarantee that you're getting exactly what you need or is in your best interest. As reports of misdiagnosis and misinformation, plus unethical practices surfacing, it's becoming increasingly hard to ignore concerns about the influence of pharmaceutical businesses on the healthcare industry.

The Business of Healthcare

One of the issues often raised is how the business of providing healthcare seems to be turning into a business driven primarily for profits, not public well-being.

This has, for instance, turned the spotlight on psychiatrists and the antipsychotics they administer to children. Did you know antipsychotic prescriptions for children increased sevenfold from the mid-1990s to the late 2000s?

In the field of psychiatry, mental illness is diagnosed based mainly on a checklist of symptoms. Scientific evidence like brain scans or blood and urine tests are not required. This can be risky especially with children who are put on mind-altering drugs while their brain is still developing. Over the years, serious and

15

irreversible complications may arise and even lead to death.

It's especially harrowing when industry insiders share their stories. Steven Francesco, a longtime executive and consultant in the pharmaceutical industry, recounts his son's journey in a memoir titled "Overmedicated and Undertreated." His son Andrew was first prescribed Ritalin when he was five to keep his rambunctious behavior until control. He became disruptive, and was given more and more antipsychotic medications as he grew older. When he was 15, one of his meds, Seroquel, resulted in a rare complication that left him brain-dead.

Gwen Olsen, a former pharmaceutical sales representative, reveals in her book "Confessions of an Rx Drug Pusher" that they were encouraged to downplay the side effects of the meds they recommended to doctors. Convinced that the drugs work, doctors prescribe those meds to their patients and those patients, Olsen says, end up being test subjects.

Practices and Priorities

Besides misinformation, the pharmaceutical industry has come under fire for a number of practices.

In terms of clinical trials, the list includes pressuring doctors to no speak about problems encountered during a study; tampering with methodology to highlight positive results; testing on people without their permission or approval; overpricing of drugs that successfully pass human trials; and bias in the reporting and publishing of outcomes.

Under-reporting of side effects, for instance, may have had a hand in the adverse reactions experienced by hundreds of women who took Bayer's birth control pills Yaz and Yasmin, both of which contain a hormone (drospirenone) that raises blood clot risk by 150% to 300%. There are in fact a number of deaths linked to the use of Yaz and Yazmin and most are due to blood clots.

Under scrutiny as well are the ties pharmaceutical businesses share with medical publishers and associations. Companies have been known to sponsor industry-related studies, which immediately casts doubt on the accuracy of the findings presented to the public. The pharmaceutical industry's reach is also believed to extend to certain guidelines issued by medical associations, especially when one of the authors has commercial ties with a specific company.

In some cases, practitioners themselves find themselves under pressure to keep their business afloat. Hence the psychiatrist who accepts commissions from the manufacturers of the antipsychotic meds he or she prescribes; the surgeon who opts to operate on a patient in order to treat a disease that could easily be managed with lifestyle changes; and the ophthalmologist who offers glasses or contacts as a fix for nearsightedness without presenting myopia rehabilitation as an option.

Note though that just because your doctor doesn't recommend natural options like complementary and alternative medicine (CAM) therapy, it doesn't necessarily mean he or she is prioritizing profit over your health. Some may be wary of giving advice related to whole medical systems, biologically based practices, and mind-body and energy medicine simply because they're not trained in CAM therapy. Others may be cautious about suggesting techniques that haven't been thoroughly (or officially) studied and tested.

None of this changes the fact that doctors save lives and a lot of times pharmaceuticals play a lead role in that. Awareness about the unfortunate realities of the business is very important too. When it comes to your health, making informed decisions could make all the difference.

Chapter 2 – Living a Healthy Lifestyle

The Centers for Disease Control (CDC) reports that in the United States alone, common viral infections like the flu affect up to 20 percent of the population each year. Over 200,000 people are hospitalized due to flu complications.

Common colds, meanwhile, are contracted by millions of people. On the average, each adult will have two to three episodes of the common cold each year, as estimated by the CDC. These figures are for colds and flu alone. There's a long list of other ailments that can be acquired if people are not careful about their health.

Although there's no reason to panic, as colds and flu are easily treatable, it's more important to focus on prevention instead of cure. And there's no better way to prevent illnesses than to lead a healthy lifestyle.

With proper diet, regular exercise, and healthy habits, you can build a stronger immune defense to ward off many types of ailments from minor ones like colds and flu to more serious ones like high blood pressure, cancer, and others.

Eat Healthy

According to the U.S. Dept. of Agriculture (USDA), American adults have significantly improved in terms of diet. People are now choosing healthier options, staying away from cholesterol, sodium, and fat, and taking advantage of nutrition information available in books and on the internet. There has also been a reduction in consumption of processed meals and fast food products.

This is definitely good news since a healthy lifestyle won't be possible without a nutritious well-balanced diet. Healthy eating doesn't always come easy. It can be a challenge if your kitchen pantry is filled with sugary snacks, junk food, and processed products.

Here are some tips that will help you eat the right foods to keep yourself in the peak of health:

Eat in Moderation

This means you should consume an amount of food that's only needed by the body, and not more than that. You should learn when to stop eating, and not devour everything in sight until you are over full.

It's also important to have a well-balanced diet consisting of the correct portions of protein, fiber, carbohydrates, vitamins, minerals and even healthy fats. All these are necessary in maintaining a healthy and strong body.

Smaller portions should also be in order. Instead of eating three huge meals, it is easier for your body to digest four to five smaller meals. Another reason it's better to eat at home than in restaurants is that you can avoid those tempting oversized meals and buffets that can cause you to eat too many carbs, calories, and less desirable fats.

Eat Less Sugar

Sugar has been called the "cocaine of the food world". The Huffington Post talks about a study showing how sugar is eight times more addictive than cocaine. Lead researcher Dr. Nicole Avena (Icahn School of Medicine, Mount Sinai) explains that the foods affecting the rewards centers in the brain are those that have high levels of glycemic load, meaning these foods can cause blood sugar levels to spike.

Addiction to sugary treats is not a problem if you can replace them with the essential nutrients needed for good health. The problem is, these are empty calories. To put simply, these are calories that do not have any nutritional value. The excessive sugar consumption has also been linked to depression, diabetes, and even suicidal tendencies.

Here are some ways you can minimize sugar in your diet:

- Drink fruit juices or fruit smoothies instead of soda.

- Eat more fruits (which are naturally sweet) whenever you're craving for cakes or chocolates.

- Watch out for hidden sugar. Many food products (even those that are not sweet) are actually packed with sugar such as commercial salad dressings, bottled sauces, and canned gravy.

Eat More Fruits and Vegetables

What you should focus more on are fruits and vegetables which are packed with nutrients like vitamins, minerals and antioxidants. The recommended daily allowance for fruits and vegetables is five servings. One serving refers to half a cup of raw fruit or vegetable.

It's certainly good for you to include more fruits and veggies in your diet. And make your choices as colorful as possible. Try adding fruit to your meals, such as topping your oatmeal breakfast with blueberries or slices of strawberries (I do this regularly for my daily breakfast routine). Pair your grilled chicken lunch with a hearty bowl of salad with corn, beets, chickpeas, kidney beans, broccoli, mushrooms, or carrots. Munch on an apple or pear for snacks instead of cookies or brownies. At dinner, you can sprinkle your whole grain pasta or soup with pieces of carrots, broccoli, asparagus, or kale.

Add More Fiber to Your Diet

We always talk about vitamins and minerals, and not enough about fiber. Dietary fiber has been found to aid in weight loss, reduce risk of heart disease and stroke, and promote proper digestion and detoxification.

According to experts, we should eat at least 21 grams of fiber each day. Unfortunately, many people are not close to eating half of this recommended amount. The basic rule is: the less processed the food is, the higher its fiber content is.

Incorporating whole grains into your diet is a must. Eat whole wheat cereals, oatmeal, barley, and unprocessed rice (such as brown rice). You should also make room for more beans and nuts throughout the day. It is recommended to avoid eating refined bread (like the Wonder Bread I had as a child), white rice, and refined pastries.

Whole grains contain high amounts of antioxidants and phytochemicals that can ward off coronary heart disease, diabetes, and even certain forms of cancer. They are also rich in healthy carbohydrates that will keep you full for longer periods of time, and help stabilize your levels of blood sugar and insulin in the body.

Go for Healthy Fats

Contrary to popular belief, not all fats are bad. There are certain fats like Trans-fats that can shoot up high blood pressure levels and make you more prone to heart disease. Good fats, on the other hand, help improve your mood, tone down inflammation inside the body, and reduce risk of cardiovascular disease.

*Here are your **Good** fats:*

- Monounsaturated fats – Avocados, almonds, pecans, hazelnuts, pumpkin seeds, sesame seeds

- Polyunsaturated fats like omega 3 fatty acids – Salmon, anchovies, sardines, herring, mackerel, flaxseeds, walnuts

*Here are your **Bad** fats:*

- Trans fats – Vegetable shortening, margarine, crackers, baked pastries, fried foods, potato chips, candies, cookies or any product that contains "partially hydrogenated oil"

Minimize Salt Intake

Salt is commonly used to add flavor to food. But most people end up consuming more salt than recommended. The maximum daily allowance for sodium is one gram, which is roughly one-half a teaspoon of table salt.

Excessive salt intake is dangerous as it can increase blood pressure level as well as increase the risk of kidney disease, heart disease, stroke, and memory loss.

Here's how you can cut down on your salt intake:

- Read labels. Sodium comes in different forms so you have to watch out for its different names: sodium sulfite, monosodium glutamate (commonly known as MSG), sodium citrate, sodium benzoate, sodium caseinate, and disodium phosphate.

- Flavor your dishes with herbs, instead of using salt or other condiments that will only put your health at risk over time. It is better to use herbs and spices to flavor food, as they have antioxidants that neutralize free radical damage inside the body, making it less prone to health problems. Garlic powder, rosemary, basil, curry powder, cayenne pepper, and black pepper will make your dishes more delicious even without the use of common table salt. If you do use some salt in your cooking, start looking for natural sea salt or Kosher Salt to replace the processed table salt you have now.

- Eat more at home. Restaurants are notorious for loading up their meals with sodium to make them more palatable. If you can't avoid eating out, the least you can do is to order low-sodium meals or request your dish to be cooked without salt. I enjoy taking the family out as a break from home cooking once a week or once every two weeks. The game we play is to search for new healthy restaurants in the area so when we do eat out we can make it "almost" as healthy as when we eat at home.

More Tips for Healthy Eating

- Stop buying unhealthy foods. Processed foods like canned meat items are high in sodium, trans-fats, and cholesterol. Sugary treats are not only loaded with sugar that can destabilize blood sugar levels, but they often also come with a lot of bad fats.

Nothing in life comes easy is the old saying. The same can be true for healthy eating. The more convenient and easy to get to food is, usually the less healthy it is for you. But fruits and nuts is an easy and convenient way to eat healthy. There are many appetizing recipes that only take a few minutes of your time. The little extra effort you put into making healthy meals will certainly benefit you in the long run.

- Put healthy foods in the front line. When storing foods in your pantry or refrigerator, always put the healthier options in front so that they'll be the first ones you'll grab when you're hungry.

- Go for healthier options. Healthy eating doesn't mean that eating cannot be fun. You just have to look for healthier alternatives. Choosing plain yogurt with fresh fruit over ice cream; popcorn sprinkled with herbs rather than eating popcorn slathered with fake butter and salt; or grilled chicken breast instead of the usual fried chicken, are just a few examples of how you can make healthy choices.

Exercise Regularly

Did you know that sitting for more than four hours each day can kill you? Sedentary lifestyle is in fact the fourth most common cause of preventable death in the world.

Research has shown that physical inactivity increases the risk of many potentially fatal ailments including heart disease, diabetes, cancer, and high blood pressure. It also causes muscle degeneration, back and neck pain, osteoporosis, depression, and dementia.

Get Britain Standing explains that sitting all day shuts down the enzymes that burn fat, slows down the body's metabolism, and reduces blood flow in the legs. Needless to say, physical activity is paramount to a healthy lifestyle. Regular exercise goes hand in hand with building a healthy body and immune system to protect you from common ailments.

In addition to reducing the risk of health problems, exercise also benefits the body in the following ways:

- Increases energy levels

- Improves your mood

- Enhances sleep quality

- Reduces stress and anxiety

Many people are aware of the benefits of exercise, but most seem not to be able to lead an active lifestyle. Lack of motivation or self-confidence, lack of time, and a busy schedule are some of the reasons that keep people from maintaining a regular exercise routine. The first step to become healthier is to stop making excuses and start incorporating physical activity in your life.

Here are a few ways to make exercise a regular part of your life:

Stop Making Excuses

People have all sorts of excuses for not exercising. The most common excuses are the following:

- "I'm too busy" – Exercising doesn't have to consume your entire day. You need to find a way to squeeze just 10 or 15-minutes into your busy schedule.

- "I'm always tired" – Physical activity can actually boost your energy so if you're always feeling tired, it's important to get moving. This will make you feel refreshed and energized.

- "I'm too fat" – Instead of using this as an excuse not to exercise, use it as a way to motivate yourself!

- "I'm not athletic" – Exercise is not reserved for athletes. That's something we should all realize. Even if you've never been into sports before, there's always some type of physical activity that will suit your abilities and benefit your body.

- "Exercise bores me" – The problem is people have limited perceptions about exercise. The word "exercise" is associated primarily with gyms and treadmills. But there's a diverse array of physical activity that you can do to keep yourself in top shape. And for sure, there's something from the list below that you'll enjoy.

- "Exercise gives me pain" – Nothing can be further from the truth. Exercise actually makes the body more flexible and less prone to pains and injuries. The initial pain that you'll feel after working out may mean that you have not done proper stretching or warm-up exercises, or that your body is still adjusting but will get used to it a short while.

How Much and What Type of Exercise Do We Need?

Mayo Clinic says that according to the Department of Health and Human Services, we should all get at least 150 minutes of moderate aerobic exercise or 75 minutes of vigorous aerobic exercise in a week. A combination of both moderate and vigorous physical activity is also recommended.

Apart from this, strength training exercises should be done at least twice every week. There are no specific guidelines when it comes to the duration of this particular physical activity.

Moderate aerobic exercises include:

- Brisk walking

- Jogging

- Swimming

- Cycling on moderate terrain

Vigorous aerobic exercises include:

- Running

- Aerobic dancing

- Mountain biking

Strength training exercises include:

- Use of weight machines or free weights

- Rock climbing

National Health Services (NHS) clarifies the difference between moderate and vigorous. Moderate is when you work hard enough to increase heart rate and produce sweat. Vigorous, on the other hand, makes you breathe hard and fast with your heart rate increasing at a much faster rate.

Safety Tips for Beginners

If you haven't exercised in a long time, or if it's your first time to establish an exercise routine, be sure to keep these safety tips in mind:

- Check with your doctor – This is especially true for those with medical concerns like asthma, diabetes, high blood pressure, or heart disease. You have to consult your doctor with regards to the type and intensity of exercise that's safe and effective for your condition.

- Do warm up exercises – Skipping warm up exercises increases risk of injury during a workout. Warm up by stretching your muscles and doing a slower version of the exercise that you'll be doing. For example, if you're going to jog, warm up by brisk walking.

- Keep yourself hydrated – It's a common mistake for exercise beginners to forget about drinking water. It's a must to take in plenty of fluids when exercising especially in warmer weather.

- Do not ignore body signals – If you feel any type of pain, distress, or discomfort, take a break. If the break makes you feel better, then it means that you can resume working out. If not, you might need to have your body checked for injury.

Tips for Success

Getting started is not the most difficult part of exercise, it's maintaining a regular exercise routine. Many people don't have any difficulty beginning an exercise program. After a while though, they start to lose interest or motivation until they are back to their old sedentary ways.

Below, you'll find some practical tips on how to make exercise a consistent part of your life:

- Pick an exercise activity that makes you happy – Choose physical activities that not only suit your abilities and health condition but also your lifestyle and preferences. As many fitness experts would advise, "think outside the gym!" The gym is not the only place in this world where you can exercise. Apart from the usual running, jogging, walking, or swimming exercises, here are other activities that you might find enjoyable:

  - Zumba

  - Ballroom dancing

  - Horseback riding

  - Golf

  - Tennis

  - Rollerblading

  - Hiking and nature walks

  - Water sports

  - Gymnastics

- ➢ Martial arts

- ➢ Rock climbing, wall climbing, mountain climbing

- ➢ Fencing

- ➢ Frisbee

- Don't be too hard on yourself – Instead of formulating an exercise program that's too ambitious, start small, and slowly build up momentum. This will make it easier for you to succeed. Once you succeed with your initial program, you can gradually progress to more difficult goals.

- Make it a part of your daily routine – Like eating breakfast or going to work, make exercise a part of your daily life. It would be better if you have a schedule for your workout. This makes it easier to establish it as a regular routine than when you make it spontaneous and leave it up to fate whether you're going to exercise on that day or not.

- Reward yourself – A rewards system is an effective way to reinforce behavior. After completing a week's workout, give yourself a treat and do things that you love (get a massage, go to your favorite concert, or buy that book that you've been eyeing for a long time). Just make sure that you don't use food as a reward as this will defeat the purpose of your exercise plan.

- Turn it into a social activity – If you're the type of person that likes to socialize, then make exercise a social activity. Form a jogging club with your neighbors, attend a dance class with your friends, or go walking with a workout buddy. You can also turn exercise into a family activity. The family who exercises together, stays healthy together!!

- Sneak exercise into your daily routine – If you can't seem to stick to a structured exercise program no matter what you do, then the least you can do is to sneak physical activities into your day. Here are some ways:

  ➤ Do chores at a brisk pace.

- ➢ Ditch the elevator and take the stairs (at least for floors 1-5)

- ➢ Park further from your office and walk the rest of the way.

- ➢ Save up on gas by using your bicycle or scooter instead of your car.

- ➢ Walk over to your co-workers to talk to them instead of sending them a message over chat or email.

- ➢ Walk while talking on the phone.

- ➢ Jog in place, stretch, or lift hand weights while watching TV.

Unhealthy Habits to Avoid

Proper diet and regular exercise is just the foundation of a healthy lifestyle. Even if you've succeeded with these two, but you have not done anything about your unhealthy habits (e.g. smoking, drinking, & other stressful things in your lifestyle), you will still be at risk of many ailments. Enumerated below are some of the bad habits that people should try to eliminate for good.

Smoking

The World Health Organization (WHO) reports that about six million people worldwide die from diseases related to the use of tobacco. Another 600,000 people die from illnesses caused by secondhand smoking. According to the CDC, tobacco use is the "single largest preventable cause of death and disease in the United States", killing over 480,000 people every year.

The most common ailment caused by smoking is lung cancer. In fact, as NHS reveals, about 90 percent of lung cancer cases worldwide can be attributed to smoking. But the lungs are not the only organs affected. The American Heart Association states that smoking is also to blame for nearly one third of deaths from heart disease.

Apart from lung cancer and heart disease, smoking also increases the risk of the following cancers:

- Throat

- Mouth

- Esophagus

- Larynx or voice box

- Liver

- Bladder

- Kidney

- Pancreas

- Stomach

By damaging the blood vessels and affecting blood circulation, smokers are also more prone to:

- Heart attacks

- Stroke

- Cerebrovascular disease (damage of the arteries supplying blood to the brain)

Moreover, it negatively impacts the respiratory system, causing problems like:

- Chronic obstructive pulmonary disease (COPD)

- Bronchitis

- Emphysema

- Pneumonia

To help you quit smoking, make use of this five-step process from the American Heart Association.

Step # 1 – Set a quit date

Within a week, designate a day when you will stop smoking. The days before this should be used for preparing yourself and slowly cutting down the number of sticks that you puff each day. Sign a no-smoking contract with your loved ones or colleagues if you think it will help you.

Step # 2 – Select method for quitting

Your first option is the "cold turkey" method, which means you'll quit smoking all at once. The second method entails reducing the number of sticks you smoke each day until you get to zero sticks. The third method requires the smoker to smoke a fraction of the cigarette.

Step # 3 – Think whether or not you will need medications to help you quit

Nicotine replacement medications (e.g. spray, gum, or the patch) can be used to help you quit smoking. Other medications, meanwhile, can help alleviate symptoms from withdrawal syndrome.

Step # 4 – Prepare yourself for your quit date

Prepare your body and mind for this date. Plan for temptations and distractions. Set yourself up for success.

Step # 5 – Quit smoking

Right after quitting smoking, your respiratory and circulatory systems will be in much better shape. You'll notice that you're feeling better after just few days.

Alcohol

Like smoking, alcohol is also harmful to health, causing many types of potentially life-threatening ailments. But that's not all, alcohol also shoots up the risk of physical injuries, particularly vehicular accidents.

In a report by the National Institute on Alcohol Abuse and Alcoholism (NIAAA), it states that roughly 88,000 people die from alcohol-related causes each year. Alcohol consumption is the third most common cause of preventable death in the US.

One or two drinks a day has been found beneficial in some studies but going over that limit can definitely wreak havoc on your health.

Driving under the influence of alcohol is not only illegal, it can be fatal to yourself, your passengers, and other drivers on the road.

If you can easily abstain from alcohol completely, that is good for you. If not, here are some tips to help you avoid drinking more easily:

Have the right reasons for quitting

If you're going to stop drinking because you need to save money for a certain gadget that you've been wanting to buy, don't count too much on succeeding. Once you've bought that item, you'll probably be back to your old ways. Whereas if you're quitting because you're concerned about your health and the wellbeing of your family, there's a bigger chance that you'll be able to stay away from alcohol for good.

Let family and friends know your plans

It gives you more motivation to succeed when you know that there are people supporting you, especially if these are people you care about. It will also make it easier for you to avoid temptations. Friends who invite you to parties or to clubs will understand why you're declining their invitation. This may mean a difficult task of staying away from some of your friends.

44

Stay away from temptations

It's important to keep temptations at bay when you're trying to quit alcohol. Surround yourself with people who will encourage you to quit, and avoid those who will get you usually just call you to have a "good time".

Cope with withdrawal syndrome

Understand that quitting alcohol won't be easy at first. If you are already dependent on this substance, there's a big chance that you will experience withdrawal symptoms like headaches, nausea, irritability, exhaustion, and convulsions. Taking medications to cope with these symptoms can make your journey less of a struggle.

Reward your success

As mentioned earlier, rewarding oneself is an effective way to reinforce a certain type of behavior. When you achieve success in your quest to quit, reward yourself with things that will make you happy, just never with alcohol.

Stress

Stress isn't always bad. In the short-term, it can boost adrenaline and improve performance. It can provide a jolt of energy necessary to complete a task. But chronic stress? That's a different story. Frequent and consistent episodes of stress can inflict serious harm on one's health.

Mayo Clinic provides a quick list of the harmful effects of stress:

Effects on physical health:

- Headache

- Muscle pain

- Muscle tension

- Chest pain

- Low sex drive

- Fatigue

- Sleeping difficulty

- Upset stomach

Effects on mental health and behavior:

- Anxiety

- Irritability

- Anger

- Temper outbursts

- Lack of motivation

- Poor concentration

- Restlessness

- Eating problems

- Use of alcohol or drugs

- Smoking

- Social withdrawal

According to Web MD, chronic stress can increase the risk of the following medical conditions:

- Cardiovascular disease

- Asthma

- Gastrointestinal problems

- Depression

- Diabetes

- Obesity

- Alzheimer's disease

Stress management is therefore necessary to maintain one's health. Reducing stress in your life will not only make you feel better but will also help ward off any future ailments that are threatening your wellbeing.

Some of the most effective stress reduction strategies that you can try include:

- Determine sources of stress – You can't get rid of stress is you don't know what's causing it. Identify the stressors that you have in your life, and take action. There are three things you can do about them: avoid, adapt or accept.

  Avoiding means staying away from the source of stress. Accepting means coming to terms that this particular stress can't be avoided and you just have to make peace with that. And then there's adapt, which means that you'll have to make changes in your life so that this stressor will no longer be a problem to you.

- Improve relationships - While people in your life can help you get through life's toughest challenges, they can also sometimes be a source of stress. Open communication and better understanding and empathy can lead to stronger and happier relationships. And having emotional support from family, in turn, can reduce stress levels.

According to the 2014 American Psychological Association Survey, 43 percent of people with no emotional support reports that they have increased overall stress in the past year.

- Practice deep breathing – When you're feeling stressed out, take a break and breathe deeply. Inhale slowly through your nose, with your eyes closed and your hand on your belly. Feel your breath fill your abdomen. Exhale slowly through your mouth. Do this for five minutes. What it does to your body is to slow down the heart rate and tone down blood pressure level.

- Relax your mind – APA's 2012 Stress in America survey reports that 40 percent of adults have difficulty sleeping at night because of stress. It's tough getting a shut-eye when your mind is filled with many things to worry about. Meditation can help. It counters stress by altering the neural pathways in the brain, enabling you to relax and empty your mind.

- Do yoga – Yoga is an effective stress reduction technique as it combines meditation and exercise. Meditation, as mentioned previously, can reduce stress levels. Exercise, meanwhile, soothes the mind by releasing feel-good hormones called endorphins.

- Engage in activities that you enjoy – Doing things that you love, whether it's talking with friends, watching a movie, reading a book, or traveling, can certainly help in alleviating your anxiety and apprehensions. Even when you're busy with work and other important things, you should always find time for yourself.

Sleep Deprivation

Sleeping is just as vital as breathing and eating. It's the body's way of resting and recuperating, as well as repairing any damages inflicted on the body during the day. Lack of sleep does not only cause daytime drowsiness, it also hinders the brain from functioning properly. Some of its immediate effects include:

- Lack of focus

- Irritability

- Excessive sleepiness

- Loss of balance and coordination

- Poor judgment and decision-making skills

But that's not all. According to Healthline, chronic sleep deprivation puts your health in danger as it weakens the body's immune defense, therefore, increasing the risk of many ailments including:

- Common cold

- Influenza

- Diabetes

- Heart disease

- High blood pressure

- Obesity

Lack of sleep has also been linked to the onset or progression of certain mental health problems like:

- Hallucinations

- Impulsive behavior

- Depression

- Paranoia

- Suicidal thoughts

Fortunately, there are ways to improve your sleeping patterns before sleep deprivation can take a toll on your health. Here are some techniques that you should follow:

- Get in sync with the natural rhythm of your body. Otherwise known as circadian rhythm, the body's natural sleep-wake cycle, can help you make the most out of your slumber. To establish this, you need to have a regular sleeping schedule, which means you need to sleep and wake up at the same time each day. Sticking to this schedule religiously will help you have a good quality sleep.

- Sleep in a dark and comfortable room – Light exposure has an effect on the body's melatonin. This is a natural hormone that's in charge of your sleep-wake cycle. The brain produces more of this when the room is dark. This is why, darkness makes you feel sleepy while light makes you feel more alert. Avoid using your smart phone or any other gadget while you're in bed as this will lessen the secretion of melatonin. Turn off the lights two hours before your bedtime.

- Get moving – Many studies have revealed that physical activity can help people sleep better during the night. It also has a positive effect on those who suffer from sleeping problems like sleep apnea and insomnia. Just make sure that you exercise in the morning and not when you're about to sleep.

- Cut down on caffeine – This will not only do your overall health a favor, it can also mean better sleep for you. National Sleep Foundation explains that caffeine is a stimulant that can disrupt sleep ten to 12 hours after consumption. This means that even if you don't drink it close to your bedtime, it can still make it hard for you to doze off. Eliminating caffeine from your diet or reducing intake will certainly be a good idea.

To keep diseases at bay, it's imperative to start living a healthy lifestyle. It doesn't have to be a major change overnight. It can be a series of small steps that revolve around the foundations of healthy eating, regular exercise and avoidance of unhealthy habits like alcohol, smoking, chronic stress and sleep deprivation.

Chapter 2 – Natural Home Remedies

Acne

Baking Soda, Lemon, Honey & Cinnamon

Baking soda fights acne by unclogging pores, removing dead skin cells and restoring proper pH balance of the skin. Cinnamon and honey have antibacterial and antiseptic properties that make them a practical acne remedy. Lemon juice, meanwhile, is rich in vitamin C that speeds up skin healing.

Ingredients:

- 1 tablespoon baking soda

- 1 tablespoon water

- 1 teaspoon cinnamon powder

- 1 teaspoon lemon juice

- 5 tablespoons honey

Instructions:

Mix all ingredients together. Spread mixture on your face evenly. Leave it on for five minutes before washing with cool water. Use this remedy once a week for one month or until acne disappears.

Oatmeal, Honey & Lemon

By clearing pores, exfoliating the skin and absorbing excess oil, oatmeal can help clear up acne in no time. Combine this with the benefits of honey and lemon, and you can say goodbye to skin blemishes for good.

Ingredients:

- 1 teaspoon honey

- 1 teaspoon lemon juice

- 1 cup cooked oatmeal

Instructions:

Combine all ingredients and gently massage onto your skin. Let it sit for 30 minutes. Rinse off with warm water. Repeat twice a week.

Allergies

Apple Cider Vinegar

For many years, apple cider vinegar has been used to treat allergies. It helps by cleansing the lymphatic system and minimizing mucus.

Ingredients:

- 1 teaspoon apple cider vinegar

- 1 glass of water

Instructions:

Pour apple cider vinegar into a glass of water. Drink this thrice a day.

Nettle Leaf

A natural antihistamine that effectively stops the body from producing allergy-causing histamine, nettle leaf can be taken in the form of a tincture or tea. Combine this with the soothing powers of peppermint and antibacterial properties of honey for instant allergy relief.

Ingredients:

- 1 tablespoon dried nettle leaves

- 1 cup water

- 1 teaspoon honey

Instructions:

Boil water and add dried nettle leaves. Steep for a few minutes. Remove from heat and strain using cheesecloth or a tea-ball. Add honey to sweeten.

Back Pain

Ginger

Ginger is an excellent remedy for the aches and discomfort brought by back pain. It has anti-inflammatory properties that you can take advantage of.

Ingredients:

- 1 piece fresh ginger root

- 1 quart water

Instructions:

Slice fresh ginger root and place ginger slices in a pot. Pour water. Bring to a boil and then simmer for 30 minutes. Let it cool for 20 minutes. Sweeten with honey. Drink this herbal tea once or twice a day.

Garlic Oil

Like ginger, garlic also acts as anti-inflammatory which speeds up healing of back pains.

Ingredients:

- 10 cloves garlic, crushed

- 2 ounces coconut oil

Instructions:

- Heat coconut oil in a saucepan. Fry garlic cloves until they turn brown. Strain oil. Put oil in a glass jar. Once cool, apply garlic oil on your back. Leave it on for two to three hours then take a warm bath.

Common Cold

Licorice Root, Marshmallow Root & Honey

Both licorice root and marshmallow root can sooth colds and sore throats by providing protective coating for the mucous membranes with their mucilage. Honey is an antibacterial that kills microorganisms triggering the common cold and its symptoms.

Ingredients:

59

- 1 tablespoon marshmallow root

- 1 tablespoon licorice root

- 1 cup honey

- 1 tablespoon ground cinnamon

- 4 cups water

- 1 tablespoon ginger, chopped

Instructions:

Mix all the ingredients together. Put in a saucepan. Simmer over low heat until syrup is reduced by half. Remove herbs by straining. Let it sit for 10 minutes more. Remove from heat and let cool. Put in a glass jar. Take two tablespoons of this syrup three times a day. The syrup lasts for up to three weeks when stored in the refrigerator.

Coconut Oil & Peppermint Chest Salve

The menthol in peppermint essential oil provides a cooling sensation that removes congestion caused by common cold.

Ingredients:

- 10 to 15 drops peppermint essential oil

- 1/2 cup coconut oil

Instructions:

Melt coconut oil in a pot. Remove from heat and let cool. Transfer to an airtight container. Pour the essential oils and shake well. Apply a bit on your chest and rub gently. You can also put a little under your nose to ease breathing.

Constipation

Fennel Seeds

Fennel seeds have long been used to remedy many digestive issues like bloating, irritable bowel syndrome and constipation. It helps promote smooth movement of muscles in the digestive tract.

Ingredients:

- 1 cup fennel seeds

- Warm water

Instructions:

Dry roast fennel seeds and then grind them until they turn into powder. Store the power in a glass jar. Take one-half teaspoon of fennel seed powder and put in a glass of warm water. Mix well. Drink everyday.

Figs & Almonds

Since figs are rich in dietary fiber, they can work as a natural laxative. Both fresh and dried figs can be used for treating constipation.

Ingredients:

- 2 to 3 pieces figs

- 2 to 3 pieces almonds

- 1 tablespoon honey

Instructions:

Soak figs and almonds in water for five to six hours. Grind and add a little bit of honey. Blend until it turns into a paste-like mixture.

Castor Oil

Another natural laxative that you can use is castor oil. It works by stimulating the intestines and promoting bowel movement.

Ingredients:

- 2 teaspoons castor oil

- 1 glass of fresh fruit juice

Instructions:

Take the castor oil on an empty stomach. You can drink fruit juice after taking in the oil to improve taste. Use this remedy only once in two weeks.

Cough

Honey

Honey is one of the oldest remedies used for cough. Its antibacterial properties make it effective as it kills the microorganisms triggering the cough and other allergic reactions. Honey also soothes the mucous membranes and alleviates pain and discomfort.

Ingredients:

- 1 tablespoon honey

Instructions:

Take one tablespoon honey two to three times a day. Children can take one teaspoon honey.

Babies should not be given honey as this can cause botulism.

Licorice Root Tea

To ease congestion and loosen mucus, take licorice root tea which works both as a demulcent and expectorant. It also tones down inflammation and soothes the throat.

Ingredients:

- 2 tablespoons dried licorice root

- 8 ounces water

Instructions:

- Boil water. Remove from heat. Add licorice root. Steep for 15 minutes. Drink the tea. Drink this twice a day.

Diarrhea

Yogurt

A good source of good bacteria, yogurt contains bifidobacterium and lactobacillus acidophilus that fight the bad bacteria in your gut causing the diarrhea.

Ingredients:

- 1 bowl of yogurt

- 1 banana

Instructions:

Mash banana into the bowl of yogurt. Snack on this twice a day.

Fenugreek Seeds

A good source of mucilage, fenugreek seeds have a strong anti-diarrheal effect and are therefore recommended to those suffering from this common ailment.

Ingredients:

- 1/2 teaspoon fenugreek seeds

- 1/2 teaspoon cumin seeds

- 2 tablespoons yogurt

Instructions:

Combine all the ingredients and mix well. Take this mixture thrice a day.

Flu

Lemon

Lemon's antiviral, antibacterial and anti-inflammatory powers can fight the flu virus that has invaded your body. It's rich in vitamin C that strengthens the immune system. It can also help soothe the symptoms that come with flu.

Ingredients:

- 1 lemon slice

- 1 cup water

- 1 tablespoon honey

Instructions:

Boil water. While still warm, squeeze the lemon slice into the water. Add honey. Stir. Drink lemon water three to four times a day.

Garlic

Garlic is not only loaded with nutrients that boost immune resistance, it also has powerful antibacterial, antiseptic, antifungal and antiviral properties that can combat flu and its symptoms.

Ingredients:

- 3 cloves garlic

- 1 cup water

Instructions:

Crush garlic cloves. Boil water in a pot. Remove from heat. Add the crushed garlic cloves. Steep for 10 minutes. Strain and drink slowly. Drink this tea three to four times each day.

Headache

Lavender Essential Oil

Whether inhaled or applied topically, lavender essential oil can efficiently alleviate headaches and relax your mind at the same time.

Ingredient:

- 5 drops lavender essential oil

Instructions:

Rub lavender essential oil on your temples and forehead. Massage gently. Repeat several times each day.

Peppermint Essential Oil

Also an excellent home remedy for headaches, peppermint essential oil is particularly useful for tension headaches. It works by stimulating blood flow in the body, thanks to its vaso-dilating and vaso-constricting properties.

Ingredient:

- 10 drops peppermint oil

Instructions:

Pour peppermint oil drops in a steamer with water. Inhale the steam. Do this two to three times each day.

Indigestion

Carom Seeds & Dried Ginger

Also called Bishop's weed, carom seeds are touted for their ability to soothe digestive ailments including indigestion, bloating and flatulence.

Ingredients:

- Handful of carom seeds

- 1 cup warm water

- 1 teaspoon dried ginger

- Pinch of black pepper

Instructions:

Grind carom seeds and dried ginger. Put one teaspoon on this in a cup of warm water. Sprinkle some black pepper. Drink once or twice a day.

Joint Pains

Turmeric & Ginger

These two root crops are famous worldwide for their medicinal benefits. They're both anti-inflammatory that can alleviate pains brought about by joint problems like arthritis. They are also rich in antioxidants that strengthen the immune system and ward off serious ailments.

Ingredients:

- 1/2 teaspoon ground turmeric

- 1/2 teaspoon ground ginger

- 2 cups water

- 1 teaspoon honey

Instructions:

Boil water in a pot. Add ground turmeric and ginger. Simmer for 10 to 15 minutes. Strain the powder. Add honey. Drink twice a day.

Epsom Salt

Epsom salt contains a naturally occurring mineral called magnesium sulfate, which has been found efficient in alleviating joint pains.

Ingredients:

- 1/2 cup Epsom salt

- Warm water

Instructions:

Get a large bowl. Fill it with warm water. Add Epsom salt. Stir with your fingers. Submerge affected joints into the water. Alternatively, you can add one to two cups Epsom salt in your bath water and soak for at least 15 minutes.

Nausea

Ginger

Among the many ailments that ginger can provide relief for is nausea. It does so by promoting the release of digestive enzymes that neutralize acid in the stomach. It also has phenols that work to sooth stomach tissue irritation and relax stomach muscles.

Ingredients:

- 1 ginger root

- 2 to 3 cups water

- 1 tablespoon honey

Instructions:

Slice ginger root. Boil water in pot over medium high heat. Add ginger. Let it boil for three to five minutes. Remove from heat and strain to remove the ginger pieces. Sweeten with honey. Drink slowly.

Sore Throat

Slippery Elm

Slippery elm has enough mucilage to coat the throat's lining, soothe irritation and tone down the pain and discomfort brought about by sore throat.

Ingredients:

- 1 teaspoon slipper elm (inner bark)

- 2 cups water

Instructions:

Put water in a pot and bring to a boil. Remove from heat. Add slipper elm. Steep for 15 minutes. Strain, and then drink slowly.

Salt Water

Gargling with salt water is another effective home remedy for sore throat. Salt is a natural antiseptic that not only cleanses the throat but also cuts down phlegm and tones down inflammation.

Ingredients:

- 1/2 teaspoon salt

- 1 glass warm water

- 1/2 teaspoon honey

Instructions:

Dissolve salt into the glass of warm water. Sweeten with honey. Gargle the mixture but don't swallow. Spit it out. Repeat three to four times a day.

Stomach Ache

Chamomile Tea

Since chamomile is an anti-inflammatory, it can be a practical solution for stomach aches. It can soothe the stomach lining which may have swollen due to gastritis or any other bacterial infection. It will lessen the abdominal pain and discomfort.

Ingredients:

- 2 teaspoons dried chamomile

- 2 cups water

Instructions:

Boil water in a pot. Remove from heat and transfer to your mug. Add dried chamomile and let steep for 10 to 15 minutes. Drink slowly.

Heat Therapy

Heat therapy works well for relieving stomach pains because heat helps relax and loosen cramped muscles.

What you'll need:

- 1 glass bottle

- 1 towel

- Water

Instructions:

Put water in a pot over medium high heat. Bring to a boil. Let it cool a little. Transfer water to a glass bottle. Cover bottle with towel so it won't burn the skin. Make sure that the bottle is just warm enough but not too hot. Gently press the bottle onto your belly for 10 to 15 minutes. Repeat as often as necessary to alleviate the pain.

Toothache

Myrrh

To get rid of the excruciating pain and discomfort caused by toothache, gargle with myrrh tincture. Myrrh does not only reduce inflammation, it also kills the bacteria causing the problem.

Ingredients:

- 1 teaspoon myrrh powder

- 2 cups water

Instructions:

Simmer powdered myrrh in water for 20 to 30 minutes. Strain to remove the powder. Let it cool. Add one teaspoon of this mixture to one-half cup water. Gargle five to six times a day.

Wounds, Bites and Burns

Coconut Oil

Thanks to its antibacterial and anti-inflammatory properties, coconut oil is one of the best ways to cleanse and disinfect a wound, bite or burn. It's also great for preventing infections and scars.

What you'll need:

- 1 tablespoon coconut oil

- Bandage

- Clean water

Instructions:

Clean wound with fresh clean water. Pat dry with a clean towel. Apply coconut oil. Cover the affected area with bandage. Reapply coconut oil and replace with new bandage twice a day.

Neem, Turmeric & Lime Juice

Also known as Indian lilac, neem is a great source of essential fatty acids that don't only keep the skin elastic but also speed up wound healing. It's also anti-inflammatory and antiseptic. Lime juice is rich in vitamin C that promotes formation of collagen. And turmeric is a wonderful antibacterial that can prevent infections.

Ingredients:

- 1 tablespoon neem leaves

- 1/2 teaspoon turmeric powder

Instructions:

Extract juice by grinding the neem leaves or blending them in a food processor. Get the juice and add turmeric powder to make a paste. Apply paste on the burn, bite or wound. Rinse off with warm water. Reapply the next few days until the wound heals.

Conclusion

The idea of being your own doctor may seem overwhelming or counter intuitive at first, but those who have tried this route attest to how effective, easy, and economical "personalized medicine" can be, thanks to the wealth of credible medical information that's available on the internet these days.

The approach should not take traditional doctors completely out of the picture. You still need the "Emergency Room" for that urgent care from accidents, lacerations, or broken bones. You still should consult your doctor from time to time and ask questions about your overall health, current condition or diagnosis, and treatment options. If you feel it's necessary or in case of a serious ailment, it is always a good idea to get a second or third opinion. Some Western medical practices have come under fire for being tied to pharmaceutical businesses and for being driven primarily for profit rather than the public's well-being, so it pays to be extra careful for any health-related decision you make.

In the end you know your body the best, and you and your loved ones have to live with each health decision you will make. Self-healthcare will help minimize the need for doctor's visits, and you will become to rely less on physicians and more confident in decisions towards a healthy lifestyle and natural home remedies.

To build your immune system and get your body in the best shape, remember that lifestyle changes are a must. You need to eat healthy by keeping your diet well-balanced, minimizing your intake of salt and sugar, focus on good fats, and add more fruits and vegetables to your daily diet. You need to keep moving regularly, end the excuses and start making time for aerobic and strength-training exercises in your everyday routine. Remember to avoid smoking and drinking; get adequate sleep every day; and reduce and manage your stress.

For simple and minor health problems, it is easy to learn natural treatments you can do at home. You'll be surprised at how simple it is make solutions for allergies, back and joint pain, flu, indigestion and constipation, diarrhea, headache, toothache, nausea, sore throat, nausea, insect bites and wounds. Most of the ingredients you'll need are either already sitting in your kitchen pantry or readily available in local stores.

As you'll see, being proactive about your health can do your body good in more ways than you can imagine. Medication is not always the best answer, and operations are not always the only option. Many times and with the help of this book, you can begin to matters into your own hands. Like the story I told you at the beginning of this book, if I did not take matters into my own hands, who knows if I would be here today.

Check Out Other Books

"Rebuild Your Health with a Mediterranean Diet" also by **Tammy Moore**